The Healing Option

How to Restore Balance, Renew Vibrant Health and Vanquish Pain and Illness by Activating Your Natural Ability to Self-Heal

Written by

Bob Berman, Soul 7 Founder

with Ara Wiseman,

R.H.N., R.N.C.P.

Produced by

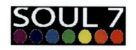

Toronto, Canada

The Healing Option ©2018 Soul 7

All rights reserved. No part of this publication may be reproduced or transmitted in any form or by any means, electronic or mechanical, including photocopying, recording, or any information storage and retrieval system, without the prior written consent of the writer or publisher, except in the case of brief excerpts in critical reviews and articles. All inquiries should be addressed to:

Soul 7 Inc.
17 Yorkville Ave., Toronto, Ontario M4W 1L1
416.847.6999 1.855.387.6857
www.soul7.ca email: info@soul7.ca

The entire content of this book is provided for informational purposes only. No part whatsoever of this book is intended as medical advice nor as a substitute for medical or other health advice. You should always consult with a medical doctor or other health care practitioner before taking any dietary, nutritional, herbal or homeopathic supplement or beginning or stopping any therapy. Readers should use their own judgment or consult with a physician or holistic health expert for specific applications to their individual problems.

When changing your diet or undergoing therapy there is always some reaction. Consequently, neither the author nor the publisher or any party responsible for the production of this book, are responsible for any adverse detoxification reactions or consequences of any kind whatsoever resulting from any information or suggestions; including product suggestions, recommendations or procedures described herein. The author has attempted to provide an understanding of the topics discussed and to ensure accuracy, however, the author and all parties associated with the production of this book assume no responsibility for errors, inaccuracies, omissions, or any inconsistencies herein.

Written by: Bob Berman, B.C.L; LL.B with Ara Wiseman, RHN, RNCP
Research assistant: Natalia Hnatiw, CNP, RNCP
Cover/interior design: Karen Thomas: Intuitive Design International Ltd.

DEDICATION

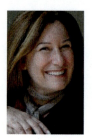

This book is dedicated to the life and memory of my high-school sweetheart and wife of 38 years, Jayne Galler Berman, whose healing love energy continues to be the source of all that is good in my life and the inspiration for Soul 7 and its Cancer Support Program.

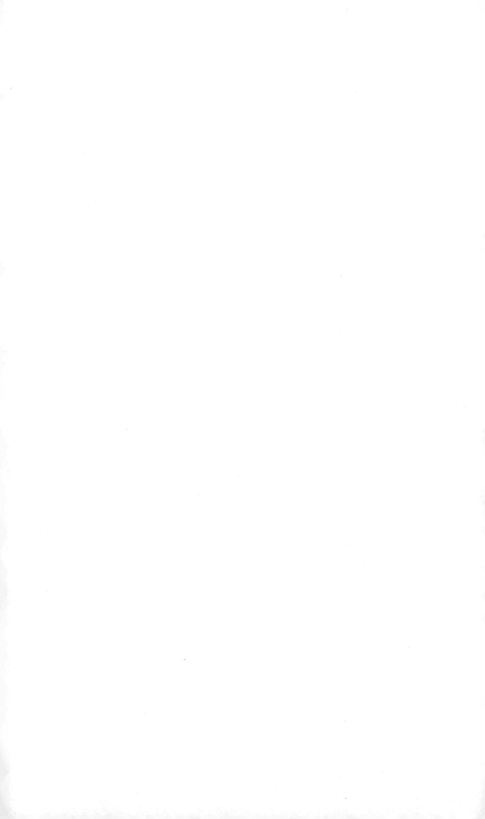

At first blink, illness – especially cancer does not look like a spiritual exercise. In the face of a serious illness, we can become paralyzed, suspend judgment and intuition and accept an environment where options seem to no longer exist. When the body is dealt a serious physical blow, doctors often take advantage of the situation, providing healing "options" that define healing within the most narrow of definitions. It is up to the individual to turn illness into a spiritual exercise and to bring dreams – and other alternative healing methods of choice – into the healing process.

– Wanda Burch from her book *She Who Dreams*

Contents

Introduction

Mission Statement

Chapter 1: Healing Power Comes From Within

Chapter 2: The Mind/Body Connection

Chapter 3: The Power of Your Subconscious Mind

Chapter 4: EMF - The Destiny Generator

Chapter 5: Technology- The Catalyst To Self-Healing

Chapter 6: Renew and Rebalance

Chapter 7: Healthy Practices

Conclusion

Introduction
The Creation of Soul 7

> Between stimulus and response there is a space. In that space is our power to choose our response. In our response lies our growth and our freedom.
>
> ~ Victor Frankl

My journey into the space between stimulus and response began about 8 years ago when my wife of 38 years developed breast cancer. When Jayne went through post partum depression after our twins were born, she became preoccupied with the notion that she was going to die at the age of 58, just like her mother. I kept telling her not to hold onto that belief. Somehow I knew that if she kept saying it, it would come true. Our thoughts and words are energy that manifest into physical form to define our reality. Jayne began to live her life anticipating her death. Paradoxically, she loved life and lived it with passion, and yet she had this strong belief that she was going to die at the age of 58.

- Our thoughts and words are energy that will manifest into physical form.

At the age of 52, Jayne developed breast cancer and needed to have a lumpectomy. Jayne was determined to live and fought back with a vengeance, choosing the extreme measure of having a double mastectomy. She then underwent extensive and debilitating reconstructive surgery on both breasts, over many months. She recovered from the surgeries quickly and everything seemed fine again, until she turned 57 when she developed abdominal pain that the doctors thought were gallstones. She continued to experience a dull pain but accepted the diagnosis.

A year later, we were told it was terminal gallbladder cancer and that she had less than two years to live. It felt like a dagger to my heart and I couldn't accept it. Jayne was ready to fight for her life, but this time there seemed to be a sense of resignation. What was happening to Jayne was devastating and would have been easier to handle emotionally if it was happening to me.

Within a few days of her diagnosis I began getting dizzy spells that I attributed to stress. Up until her diagnosis I had been in the best physical condition of my life. I was working out four times a week and

felt like I did when I was in my 20's. My heart had been checked a few months earlier and was in fine condition. With overwhelming dizziness I was admitted into the same hospital that Jayne was receiving her treatment. All the time that Jayne was researching my condition she continued dealing with her own terminal diagnosis. She was focused on my situation and I was focused on hers. Meanwhile, our children had to deal with the fact that both of their parents were in the same hospital with life-threatening health issues.

I needed immediate open-heart surgery to replace the closed valve. The heart surgeon wanted to put in a mechanical valve as it might last longer than a tissue valve. I just wanted to get the surgery done so I could start looking after Jayne. In the end the surgeon was unable to fit the mechanical valve, so he put in a valve made from pig tissue. I now realize that the dagger in my heart from Jayne's terminal diagnosis was the reason for my heart issue. To fulfill my life purpose, I needed to spiritually heal my heart and the mechanical valve wasn't energetically capable of spiritual healing. The Universe gave me the opportunity to heal and I have seized that opportunity.

After I was able to leave the hospital, I started looking into alternative healing practices for Jayne. One of them was energy healing. I had taken a course on Neuro-Linguistic Programming (NLP) at the Ontario

Hypnosis Center. NLP is a method of influencing people with words, and as a lawyer I thought it would be a helpful approach to study. I became a master practitioner and began using it in my law practice. One day, the Ontario Hypnosis Center was advertising Energy Healing. It sparked my interest and I thought it could help Jayne.

This is when I first met Dr. Sharon Forrest, an energy healer from Vancouver who was brought in through the Ontario Hypnosis Center. Jayne was hesitant but agreed to try it for me. Jayne responded positively to it and felt that it was helpful. Unfortunately, Dr. Forrest resided in British Columbia and informed us that we would have to continue remotely over Skype. Remote healing over the Internet was too much for Jayne to accept, so she didn't continue. I started looking into alternative healing practices, which led me to reading the works of Dr. T Collin Campbell and Dr. Caldwell Esselstyn. We met with Dr. Esselstyn at the Cleveland Clinic and went on a vegan diet for a short period of time.

Like most of us, Jayne believed in conventional medicine and was of the mindset that her doctors knew best. At that time, the doctors were suggesting chemotherapy followed by surgery in order to extend her life without actually curing her. We consulted with a doctor in the US and he suggested surgery without chemo, which in hindsight would have been the right choice. Unfortunately, in Ontario, in order to qualify for the expensive, radical surgery that Jayne needed, there had to be a favorable reaction to the chemotherapy. The medicare system uses chemotherapy as a filtering mechanism, because chemotherapy is less expensive then surgery. I found out after Jayne had the surgery that if she had not responded to the chemo, the surgery that she desperately needed would not have been made available to her.

Jayne responded to the chemotherapy, but it left her immune system too weak to recover from the surgery. She had rushed the surgery in order to be able to attend our oldest son's wedding in Edmonton. Right before the wedding, Jayne had a mild stroke but was still determined to go. We took the train from Toronto to Edmonton to avoid air travel. The day of the wedding, Jayne was re-energized and glowing with happiness. By the time the evening was over Jayne began to unravel. We ended up in the hospital and soon after we flew back to Toronto. I continued to look into alternative therapies but Jayne was too weak to try anything else. Despite having an enormous will to live, Jayne died just a few days later at the age of 58, just as she had predicted.

About a month after her death, I began receiving calls from Dr. Forrest, the energy healer that Jayne and I had seen. Upon hearing the news of Jayne's death, she insisted I join her on her annual trip to Peru to do volunteer work. I declined, but the Universe had other plans for me. Dr. Forrest had been receiving "messages" that it was important that I go to Peru. So next thing I knew, I was in Lima with Dr. Forrest and sixteen women, all energy healers.

About 3 hours out of Cusco, I was sitting on a bus thinking sadly about Jayne. Lisa who was sitting beside me, tapped me on the shoulder and told me she kept getting a persistent message for me from someone who had passed. She asked me if the name Sophia meant anything to me. I was relieved because the name had no relevance. She looked puzzled but as I thought more deeply about it, I realized that it was my daughter's middle name. She told me that she was referring to someone much older. Suddenly, it dawned on me that this was also Jayne's grandmother's name. Lisa then proceeded to tell me that my wife was fine and not to worry about her. How did she know? As soon as we arrived at the village I asked Dr. Forrest if she had told anyone about my story and my recent loss, and she assured me that she hadn't. This was the beginning of my spiritual awakening and transformation.

On the third day of my journey I met a Shaman named Roberto who only spoke Spanish. Up to this point I wasn't even sure what a Shaman was. We shared a room and spent a lot of time together on side trips to waterfalls and wildlife areas. On these walks, I found myself drawn energetically to certain stones and rock formations. I would kneel down and feel the earth's energy. While on a walk, I became very sad and separated myself from the group. Roberto seemed to appear out of nowhere and began doing a ritual on me that involved moving his hands around my head and body and spraying me with water from his mouth. He then directed me towards a path up the mountain where a blue and white butterfly materialized and followed me for the next hour. I felt Jayne's presence in that butterfly and this gave me peace of mind. When I reached the bottom of the mountain I felt the earth's energy flow through me and I fell to my knees. This was my first energetic experience.

During a visit to Machu Picchu, Roberto took me to a sacred rock carved by the Incas that was off limits to tourists. He performed another ritual on me, which led me to have an out of body experience. I was soaring above the clouds with a feeling of ecstasy. White light surrounded me and I was at peace. Eventually, I felt the sensation that I was being pulled back down into my body and I woke up to an enormous centipede on my leg, which I later found out, is a sign of spiritual awakening.

In the months that followed my return to Toronto, I became certified in crystal healing and hypnosis. I was drawn to European alternative cancer therapies that I thought might have worked for Jayne. I realized that my mission was to help others to heal. I wanted to open people up to the idea that there is healing energy within each and every one of us. I decided to use the European healing tech-nologies that I had discovered, in order to help people become aware of and access their body's innate healing wisdom. This led me to the opening of Soul 7, a healing centre that combines ancient healing wisdom with state-of-the-art alternative healing technologies.

Jayne's passing left me devastated. It has also taught me that death is a new beginning, a time for healing. It has led me to a burning desire to help people tap their own innate ability to heal themselves and reach their optimal health, whatever that may be. Everything is energy and as Einstein, said "Energy is neither created nor destroyed."

I believe that death simply transmutes energy from this life to the next and that's where Jayne's energy is right now, waiting for her next life and making sure my children and I live our lives to our optimal health ... which is my wish for you.

– Bob Berman, Founder

Our Mission
Soul 7

We believe that every person has the ability to heal...

Soul 7's mission is to introduce people to and help optimize their innate ability to Self Heal by combining the metaphysics of ancient healing wisdom with the quantum physics of sound, light and electro-magnetic frequency technologies. We call this combination Mindful Healing Technologies

Chapter 1

Healing Power Comes From Within

> The doorway to perfect health opens inward.
>
> ~ Fabrizio Mancini

The body's natural inclination and wisdom is to always strive for health and balance—it knows exactly what it needs in order to heal itself. The healer is within each of us. The problem is that most of us have lost this intuitive connection and need to reconnect to this intelligence. We live in an external world and look to external sources for everything. External sources are only there to remind our body to reconnect to this inner healing wisdom. Our false beliefs are what get in the way of healing, often causing us to feel powerless and vulnerable.

According to Patti Conklin, Ph.D., the word FEAR stands for Forgetting Every Available Resource. We need to just step back, release the fear and trust and have faith that every resource is already inside us. When we are in fear we can't see the forest for the trees and lose hope and faith in our body's ability to heal itself. Fear triggers the release of stress hormones, shutting down our innate healing mechanism, triggering left-brain dominance and keeps us searching externally for the answers. We experience pain and sickness because we are not listening to the subtle messages from our bodies. We may intuitively know but not always listen, because we might have to make a change to our current situation, and that produces fear. In the movie Crazy, Sexy Cancer, Kris Carr says, "fear is the cancer." Nothing is insurmountable. We just have to bring our physical, emotional and spiritual body back into alignment in order to be able to access our innate healing wisdom.

We can access our body's natural healing wisdom when we are in a state of love, appreciation, gratitude and serenity. Every thought we experience produces an effect in our body at the cellular level. Our cells communicate with each other by means of wavelengths (frequencies). When we are thinking, our cells are listening and releasing neuropeptides (chemical signals) in response to our thoughts, affecting the functioning of our immune system and every cell in our body. A toxin or toxic thought is a disorganized frequency pattern that interferes with our body's natural functions. My mission at Soul 7 is to use our Mindful Healing Technologies to transform the frequency patterns that cause illness, into therapeutic healing frequencies that restore the body's equilibrium. When we are feeling frustrated, stressed, defeated and unhappy, we are in the fight or flight response and our bodies innate healing mechanism is shut off. In order to heal, we must be in a homeostatic state, feeling relaxed and balanced. In this relaxed state we release hormones like dopamine, oxytocin and endorphins that are healing to the body.

When faced with an illness, it is difficult to not stress out over it—this is only natural. According to ancient wisdom, the solution exists before the problem is created. Unfortunately, we can't always see it because we are in a state of fear and disbelief. With Mindful Healing Technologies, we now have access to self-healing that we could never have dreamed possible. This state of the art technology stimulates and facilitates your body's innate healing mechanisms. These unique stress reduction therapies include, guided visualization, sound and light technology, and brain wave modulation. These therapies help to create feelings of hope and optimism, and a relaxed state of calm giving you the ability to focus inward and access your body's own healing wisdom. According to Charlotte Gerson, "Cancer is totally curable by restoring the body's ability to reactivate this healing mechanism." When we provide our body with optimal living conditions and surround ourselves with a nurturing environment that is healing both physically and emotionally, we can begin to heal. Healing comes from within, but sometimes we need help accessing it.

Mindful Healing Technologies can be a catalyst to the healing energies within each of us. Even though healing is a personal journey, it doesn't have to be done alone. The body is a marvelous creation, always striving to bring itself back into balance. When given the right support, recoveries that are deemed 'miraculous' can become common and the incurable can become curable. We all have it within us.

> You can't keep one disease and heal two others.
> When the body heals, it heals everything.
> ~ Charlotte Gerson

Self-healing allows us to become active participants in our own lives in order to further our physical, mental and spiritual understanding and their inter-relationship. When we understand the purpose of disease and its underlying root cause, we can see it as a process of transformation and live more fully with insight and awareness, ultimately developing a deeper relationship with ourselves. When the purpose of disease is understood, our level of consciousness shifts enabling us to see the disease as the first step towards health and balance—not just random circumstance.

Do you know that you have healed yourself millions of times since birth through the body's natural healing system? It is never too late to make changes. Your body is forgiving and renewable. Your cells are constantly renewing and repairing and every seven years you have a completely new body. The skin covering your body is only about four weeks old, your stomach lining is about five days old, your liver is five months old and your bones are about ten years old. In fact, ten to twenty billion cells throughout your body die everyday and are replaced. Our natural inclination is to change, create and grow.

> All the illness that afflicts people comes only because of a lack of joy....
>
> And joy is the great healer.
>
> ~ Rabbi Nachman

The more complex the diseases are, the more indicative they are of the layers of emotions that have been stored. Unresolved, unexpressed emotions are tucked away in our body, hidden from our conscious awareness. We need to dig deep inside to get to the root, back to the seed level of when it was first planted. It could be a childhood trauma rooted in our distant past or an unresolved sadness, anger or unexpressed resentment. I believe that the stages of cancer, for example, represent the deep roots and layers of these emotions and how intensely they have been affecting us. For instance, stage four cancer, is an indication of how deeply imbedded in our tissues the unresolved issues are. It is a seed that was planted that has been growing inside and needs to be dealt with.

Dr. R.G. Hamer discovered that a biological conflict strikes on three levels simultaneously: the psyche, the brain and the organ. He found that breast cancer has its origins in different areas of the brain, resulting from a conflict or trauma. "Since breast gland cancer has its origin in the cerebellum, or old brain, the tissue starts to augment from the time of the onset of the actual conflict, and will stop growing as soon as the conflict has been resolved."[1]

> When emotions are expressed all systems are united and made whole. When emotions are repressed, denied, not allowed to be whatever they may be, our network pathways get blocked, stopping the flow of the vital feel-good unifying chemicals that run both our biology and our behavior.
> ~ Candace Pert

As we go through our lives and experience ordinary daily conflicts, it is normal to experience a full range of emotions. These day-to-day conflicts are different than the continuous stress we experience from deep internal conflicts. Diseases don't always manifest because we are having an internal conflict. It is only when we are in a prolonged stress phase that specific symptoms and imbalances are caused that lead to disease. If you had a chain and you kept stressing the chain, eventually it would break. When we get emotionally stressed, we all have an area in our bodies that is more prone to being affected. The nature of the conflict we tend to experience will repeat itself until we figure out what the message represents. It is during this 'aha' moment of realization that we experience a shift in our consciousness and we are given what we need to resolve it. It's interesting to note that each organ has a corresponding emotion that the nature of the conflict relates to. This is the area in our body where the pain will be felt or where the disease will manifest. Sometimes it is in the resolution or shealing phase that we begin to feel the physical symptoms. For example, when you are going through a stressful event in your life, it is usually after the event has passed that you end up exhausted mentally and physically. According to Candace Pert, Ph.D., "Our mind is in our body and our body is our subconscious mind."

We don't have to be happy all the time in order to be healthy. Being emotionally healthy is about allowing our feelings to come up, feeling them and then letting them go, so that the past isn't being carried over to the present. When you let go of the need to control things in your life—your attachment to the outcome of things—you move into a state of neutrality and are able to accept whatever may happen next. Not being limited by your past experiences creates freedom and allows for expansion. Usually, when we experience fear or stress, we contract our energy and end up with pain or other symptoms. My goal for Soul 7's advanced technologies is to allow you to move your awareness out of resonance with your negative thoughts and emotions by helping you access a state of balance and neutrality, opening you up to an infinite sea of Healing Options that already exist around you.

---

[1] http://www.newmedicine.ca

Chapter 2
The Mind/Body Connection

> Disease and disharmony appears in the mind before it appears in the body.
>
> ~ Dr. Christine Page

I have found in my journey with my wife and especially since her passing, that one of the benefits of suffering, including illness, is that it can begin the process of questioning, seeking and striving to understand ourselves. In that process, we can begin to grasp the notion that our mind and body are one and that we have an innate healing wisdom inside.

Our bodies do not only metabolize food, they also process emotions. In the Western culture, we have been taught to believe that the mind is in the head. In fact, the mind manifests itself in the body. Thoughts and emotions are capable of creating harmony or disharmony. The power of the mind and the emotions affect the overall health of the body by affecting the immune and nervous systems. Thoughts create neuropeptides and every cell in our body has a neuropeptide receptor. Therefore, when we are thinking, our cells are listening. It is interesting to note that the neurotransmitters present in our brain are also present in our gut, which is why it is considered our 'second brain.' This explains why we often have what is known as 'a gut instinct' about something. We need to learn to trust that instinct and listen to our body's wisdom.

According to Candace Pert, PhD., "Thoughts and emotions bubble up from the body to the brain, where we can process and verbalize them according to our expectations, beliefs and other filters—some get through and others don't." The problem lies in the fact that we all have conditioned thoughts and beliefs about everything and can't always hear the messages our body is giving us. Oftentimes, when we are dealing with an illness or life-changing event, we may try to deny feelings of stress or fear. It is important to feel every feeling you experience—even the negative ones—and to not feel guilty for having those valid feelings. Allow yourself to experience a wide range of emotions. Don't judge them. Let them go. *The key to the Healing Option is to allow ourselves to fully release negative feelings and transform them into gratitude for everything we have.*

No matter what life hands us, we all have thousands of things we can be grateful for. One of the most important things you can do in your life is to "be here now." Slow down physically and mentally—and take a breath, smell the roses. Turn off your cell phone, computer, all your devices, and just pause.

> Consciousness isn't just in the head. Nor is it a question of the power of the mind over the body...because they're flip sides of the same thing. Mind doesn't dominate body, it becomes body.
>
> ~ Candace Pert

I created Soul 7 to introduce technologies that can help immerse you into a receptive state that allows you to hear what your mind is trying to tell you. When we reach deep levels of relaxation we create within us the ideal condition that is needed to focus our mind in order to send healing messages to our body and to strengthen new thought patterns.

> Remember the master program in the subconscious must be changed before the circumstances will change.
>
> ~ Karol K. Truman

According to DeAnn Gershbein, an energy healer in Vancouver, "Whenever a traumatic event in your life occurs, all the psychological, emotional and physical aspects that are connected with it are contained within that memory." For example, if you have been in a car accident, driving down the same street where it happened can re-trigger the initial trauma and shock, causing it to resonate throughout your body. The original injury and pain, even if it has healed, may still be felt along with the memory because it has been recorded in your subconscious. The memory always remains but the trauma can be released and removed. You can clear the trauma from the memory and then the memory no longer has any pain associated with it.

Since Jayne's passing, I have come to realize that releasing trauma is a critical part of healing. I have learned through my research that Guided Visualization, a form of self-administered hypnosis, can help to access the subconscious level where the trauma of the memory has been stored and begin to heal the trauma and change your thoughts associated with that memory.

And that brings me to the placebo effect and spontaneous remission...

According to Caryle Hirshberg, "Spontaneous remission is the disappearance, complete or incomplete, of a disease or cancer without medical treatment or by treatment that is considered inadequate to produce the resulting disappearance of disease symptoms or tumor."

There are thousands of incurable illnesses that have miraculously healed through the power of the mind. It is our expectation, belief and subconscious trust, not only in the pill or treatment but also in the person administering it. We expect to feel better and our subconscious mind is in line with that belief, which activates the immune response, thereby releasing pain relieving endorphins. When a child gets hurt and you give them a bandage they often feel better. It doesn't fix the cut or scrape, but it provides reassurance and comfort for the child. The mind is so powerful that we can manifest what we believe. In Anthony Robbin's book, *Unlimited Power*, he describes a woman who had a split personality. One of her personalities was diabetic while the other was not. Her blood sugar would be normal when she was in her non-diabetic personality, but when she shifted into her diabetic alter ego, her blood sugar rose, and all medical evidence demonstrated that she was diabetic. When her personality flipped back to the non-diabetic counterpart, her blood sugar normalized.

What makes our beliefs so powerful is the effect they have on every cell in our body. Mr. Wright, a man who suffered from a rare form of cancer, is another example of the power of the mind. After exhausting all possible treatment options he was given only a week to live.

However, news of a new miracle drug being offered in clinical trials gave him hope. He knew he didn't want to die and convinced his doctor to let him try the drug. Within a few days of his first dose, he was feeling better and his tumors miraculously shrunk to half their original size. Just ten days after receiving the drug, he was cancer-free and out of the hospital. Unfortunately, the story doesn't end there. Reports surfaced two months later that the miracle drug he was given was deemed to be ineffective. Upon hearing the news, he became very depressed and his cancer returned. Mr. Wright's doctor realized what was happening and convinced him that he would give him a better version of the drug, that was sure to cure his cancer. Although he injected him with nothing more than distilled water, the tumors began to disappear. Mr. Wright believed that he was getting the best treatment from his doctor and this belief was healing his body. Once again, the American Medical Association announced that the so-called miracle drug was completely ineffective and Mr. Wright lost all hope in the treatment. His cancer came back and he died a few days later.

Our beliefs manifest and produce lasting results when we reach that place deep within, at the core of our being, knowing without a shadow of a doubt what is going to happen next. The opposite of the placebo effect is the nocebo effect, in which we manifest our negative thoughts, becoming a self-fulfilling prophecy. When we think something bad is going to happen to us, and constantly live in fear of it, we are inviting it into our lives. We even begin to live our lives in anticipation of it. When a doctor tells us the negative side effects of a medication, it is the power of suggestion and our belief and anticipation of it happening that creates a self-fulfilling prophecy. For example, if a doctor tells his patient that he is likely to feel nauseous or get a headache from a medication, he most likely will, even if it's a sugar pill. Patients who were given saline injections while thinking that it was chemotherapy, threw up and lost their hair.

When you give or receive a hug healing hormones are released. Serotonin, dopamine and endorphins, our feel good neurotransmitters, flood your body. That warm feeling you experience is from oxytocin, also known as the cuddle hormone. When we connect with others we let go of our sense of separateness, sending healing signals to our brain. During the embrace, our solar plexus chakra gets activated and stimulates our thymus gland, improving our immunity. Hugging is healing for your heart and soul, so...don't be surprised if you receive a hug from me, or one of our Soul 7 staff before and after your session!

As you can see, the power of the mind can produce profound effects on our bodies and overall health. This is why it is so important to have a positive mindset in order to be healthy. The mind and body are intimately connected to each other. Both are also dependent on the earth's healing frequency, 7.83 Hz, known as the Schumann Resonance. That's why all of the therapies at Soul 7 incorporate this frequency. This creates a relaxed peaceful state of mind, producing positive neuropeptides and hormones helping to harmonize your mind and emotions and open you up to a whole new realm of possibilities, where your Healing Option can be fully engaged.

I believe that all disharmonies in the body are messages telling us that something is out of alignment and needs attention. Each and every one of us has a different area in our life that requires change in order to restore balance. Disease helps us move forward as it is a personal journey to understand ourselves on a deeper level by forcing us to look within. It's a wake up call—a call to begin to make the necessary changes in our lives. I believe that everything happens for a reason and that nothing is random. Sometimes we have to take the long and winding road to arrive at the place in our lives where we are meant to be. There is an expression that, 'when we are ready the teacher will come.'

The teacher is within you. You have only to look inward with faith and trust to find your personal healing option.

Chapter 3

The Power of Your Subconscious Mind

Are you continuously feeling overwhelmed and stressed? Do you feel stuck? Would you like to achieve more in your life? Are you currently suffering from any pain or disharmony in your body? What subconscious beliefs do you think may be getting in your way? Tapping into the power of your subconscious mind can transform your life.

- What is the subconscious mind?

> You are a more a product of your thoughts, than your genes.
> – Bruce Lipton

The subconscious mind is a collection of everything you have seen, heard and experienced throughout your lifetime. Whether you are aware of it or not, all of your thoughts, beliefs, experiences, impressions, images, memories, and desires have been stored in your subconscious mind. Any thought that comes to you through your five senses gets classified, recorded and stored in your subconscious. It becomes our map and how we model our reality. It is what motivates us, gives us our sense of right and wrong, and shapes our values and self-image. It influences a lot of what we do throughout our day.

Have you ever been driving and found yourself lost in your thoughts, only to discover that you had travelled miles down the road? It was your subconscious mind that was driving the car successfully during that time. Have you ever automatically taken your route to work on your day off when you were heading somewhere else? When our conscious mind is busy exploring new thoughts, our subconscious mind is helping us conduct our lives.

In the movie *The Eternal Sunshine of the Spotless Mind*, Jim Carrey's character wants to have his memories of a past relationship deleted, but instead his entire subconscious mind gets erased. As it is being erased, he sees fragmented images of everything he experienced throughout his life. He was desperately trying to hold on to his memories, realizing that they were a meaningful and important part of him. Our memories and experiences are woven into the fabric of who we are. Our subconscious can be likened to a filing cabinet that stores everything we have experienced.

When you are making a decision, your subconscious will reveal experiences and beliefs that correspond with that decision. We consciously choose what we want, but our subconscious mind is the implementer. Therefore, it is important to align what you want in your conscious mind with what you believe in your subconscious mind. According to Candace Pert, PhD, our body is our subconscious mind, as all of our emotions, traumas, memories and information are stored in it.

Your thoughts, feelings, attitude and mood affect the overall health of your body by activating chemical switches that regulate gene expression. The emerging science of Epigenetics is discovering that only a small percentage of diseases are genetic. When adopted children are raised in a family with a history of cancer, they have the same probability as biological children of developing cancer.[1] According to Bryant A. Meyers, "Genes are no longer deterministic, they are only potentials." With the right thoughts, beliefs, perceptions, diet, water, air and electromagnetic energy from the earth, we can influence how our genes are expressed.

Our subconscious is very sensitive to our thoughts and accepts that which we believe. It doesn't reason things out like our conscious mind, so what we are habitually thinking gets stored. Our conscious mind is awake and aware of our physical existence and our feelings and emotions, and makes choices based on our perception of what is happening. These perceptions are influenced by the past experiences, beliefs, programming and conditioning that we have accumulated throughout our life and are stored in our subconscious mind. Our perceptions and thoughts create our beliefs, which result in our experiences. What we think about, we bring about. We create and shape our lives with our thoughts.

Our subconscious is always listening to the input from both our conscious and higher conscious mind. Carl Jung, the Austrian Psychoanalyst, referred to our higher conscious mind as the super-conscious mind and felt that the collective wisdom and knowledge of the ages was contained in it and available to everyone. Our super-conscious mind is the innermost place of knowing, the infinite field of potential without boundaries or limitations. It has also been referred to as the universal subconscious mind or the collective unconscious. It can be likened to the internet, the gateway to seemingly endless information. All the great inventors, artists, composers and writers have tapped into their super-conscious mind, as it is the source of pure creativity.

The subconscious mind is the intermediary between the conscious and superconscious, the bridge between the individualized human self and the higher self. Most of us think that our conscious mind is the most powerful, but it is not. When we are making decisions, there are countless things that are going on simultaneously, as we are thinking on many levels in a parallel way. Understanding how your mind operates will help you manifest a happier and healthier life by connecting to your higher consciousness.

Imagine if you could access your higher consciousness. Imagine if you could to understand why you had chosen to go through painful and joyful experiences, while at the same time discovering your life purpose and what you need to do in order to achieve it. I want you to open yourself up to the possibility that you can. I assembled Soul 7's revolutionary technologies to help bypass the conditioned beliefs that are subconsciously stored in our minds. Together, these technologies help to access a deep and flowing state of healing energy that activates the body's immune system to induce self-healing.

Inspiring thoughts and ideas often come to us when we are sleeping, because we are not operating from our conscious mind where there may be self imposed limitations based on fear (False Evidence Appearing Real). When we are asleep we are in a different brain wave frequency that allows us to be more relaxed and creative. Have you ever noticed that when you are inspired and excited to achieve something in your life, there is a continuous flow of ideas and you have the energy needed to facilitate that goal? It is like plugging into the universal energy outlet. We are continuously evolving in our awareness and our ultimate goal is to align and connect with the universal or higher consciousness.

> Before you can inspire with emotion, you must be swamped with it yourself. Before you can move their tears, your own must flow. To convince them, you must yourself believe
>
> ~ Winston Churchill

- How can I harness the power of my subconscious mind?

Understanding the relationship between the conscious and subconscious mind can transform your life. Our subconscious can either be a bridge or a barrier to manifest our desires. When we have a desire to make changes in our lives and we think about it consciously without believing and feeling it deeply within, it won't manifest. Our subconscious mind holds on to our past experiences and previously held beliefs about ourselves. Keep in mind that a lot of the thoughts that are running through your mind are unconscious and you are creating your reality with your thoughts and beliefs. Our subconscious doesn't have the ability to correct any of our illogical or irrational beliefs. It is like a computer that holds everything we put into it, so we have to reprogram it to change our internal beliefs about ourselves. Our subconscious is the part of the mind that bridges our outer self with our spiritual self, as it listens to the input from our conscious and our higher consciousness. Our higher consciousness wants us to evolve and pushes us in a new direction. Holding on to the past, being afraid of change and wanting everything to remain the way it is, oftentimes will result in emotional distress or inner turmoil. The goal is to minimize or eliminate the subconscious barrier and create a bridge from the physical world to our higher self.

You might have heard the expression 'you need to believe it first before you see it,' but what exactly does that mean? In order for us to manifest our desires, we need to feel it deep inside, believe it, and envision the reality we prefer as already existing in the present moment. How would you feel or live your life differently if you had met your soul mate or were living a life without pain or illness? We need to match the frequency of what we wish to receive by living our lives as though our desires have already been attained. Breathe life and energy into your thoughts through your feelings. When we want to change something in our lives, we can acknowledge what exists presently while inviting in a new possibility from the infinite field of possibilities. The more intense your feelings are, the more powerfully you activate that version and the more quickly it manifests into your tangible reality. I know you are probably thinking, easier said than done. Well, that would be your subconscious mind revealing your conditioned limitations of what you believe to be possible. You need to reprogram your software in order to realize the infinite potential that exists around you. The Mindful Healing Technologies that I have synergistically combined can help you do this by releasing negative energy from your subconscious and creating more space for the positive energy of the new possibilities that already exist.

Whether we are consciously aware of them or not, we all have experiences that are affecting us physically. My exploration of the ancient healing wisdoms of Peru, has taught me that every thought that we have sends a frequency out into the universal matrix, which is full of every possibility coexisting simultaneously. We can influence this field with our heart and through our feelings. Our heart has a strong electromagnetic field, creating waves that influence the world around us. We can't just intellectualize our desires we need to feel them. The problem is that most of us think about the things we don't want and have an emotional reaction to it, which ends up bringing us more of what we don't want.

Our natural state is to grow and change, but sometimes we get stuck. Maybe your self-perceptions, current relationships, or how you have been living your life up until now, no longer supports the person you are today or the person you wish to become. You need to reprogram your outdated perception of yourself to match the person you are today. We do this by letting go of what no longer serves us. When our body and emotions are in a balanced receptive state, our higher consciousness is more accessible.

Our physical reality, where we are presently in our lives, is a mirror, a reflection of what we most strongly believe to be true. Every day is a new opportunity for Self Awareness- the knowledge of what beliefs need to Change to begin to optimize your ability to Self Heal. We choose The Healing Option when we have the Courage to act on that Self Awareness. What would your life look like if you had Self Awareness and acted on it?

> Feeling is the union of thought and emotion.
>
> ~ Gregg Braden

For thousands of years, man has used prayers or affirmations to communicate desires. Prayers that appear to go unanswered are the result of a subconscious mind overwhelmed by negative thoughts and energy. When you pray or affirm, what is going through your mind?

Are you thinking about your to-do-list, what to cook for dinner or a problem you are dealing with at work?

There is a story of a Rabbi who would greet his student's everyday before prayers as if they had just come back from a vacation and hadn't seen them for a while. One of his students wanted to know why. He explained that it was intended to remind them to be present in their prayers. Oftentimes our minds wander and we are not present in what we are doing; it's as if our mind has gone on a mini vacation. Prayers and affirmations aren't just words, they are feelings. The words are there to direct our intention but it is our feelings that inject it with life and energy. When you are praying or repeating affirmations, it is important to be mindful of your thoughts and be clear about your intention. Your desires may not be manifesting because, like most of us, you are not able to stop negative thoughts, self-talk and programmed beliefs from seeping into your mind. Our desires either harmonize or conflict with our core beliefs, which are stored in our subconscious.

There is a famous expression by Richard Bach, "change the way you see things and the things around you will change." How can you realistically do this when you are experiencing approximately 60,000 thoughts per day, and you are not even consciously aware of most of them? It takes practice, patience and can be facilitated with the right technology.

In my journey that led to the birth of Soul 7, I found that technology may be a great way to reprogram your subconscious by altering your brainwaves through sound and light. It induces a brainwave frequency equal to 7.83 Hz that is aligned with the earth's pulsating magnetic field and the vibrational frequency produced by chanting the OM sound. It's interesting that if you rearrange the letters in the word 'earth' you get 'heart.' The earth is a living organism and its heartbeat is approximately 7.83 Hz, which is also known as the Schumann Resonance Frequency. Every living thing is tuned to the earth's pulse. We have a body-mind-earth connection to the frequencies the earth emits. Our tissues and cells absorb them, our brain is tuned into them and we even emit them. Our cells respond to this frequency and our nervous system and brain are tuned into it, which is why it is so calming and healing. This frequency is the gateway to deeper states of consciousness. When we are in deep meditation we go from Alpha to Theta brainwave frequencies. It is in these frequencies that we are able to access our higher consciousness and the infinite field of potential. In this relaxed, receptive state we can change our perceptions and become aware of our subconscious thoughts in order to begin reprogramming them. Mindful Healing Technologies are designed to positively influence your thoughts, reprogram your subconscious and set the tempo to activate your healing option.

---

[1] PEMF, The 5th Element of Health, Bryant A. Meyers, © 2014, Bryant A. Meyers

Chapter 4

EMF:
The Destiny Generator

> We each broadcast energy that will determine its own consequences,
> thus becoming the generators of our own destiny.
>
> ~ Author Unknown

- What is energy?

Everything and everyone, including you, is made up of atoms that emit waves of energy called electro-magnetic frequencies (EMF). Atoms continuously give off and absorb light and energy and have their own unique frequency and vibration. The energy is continuously moving in waves; where one atom stops another begins. It is constantly flowing and changing form and doesn't even stop when you are asleep. Our cell's membrane has an electrical charge that creates impulses and sends messages through electrical signals around the body. Every cell emits energy, creating an electromagnetic energy field that can also be measured outside of your body. Therefore, we are interacting energetically with everyone around us and with nature, in the electromagnetic fabric of our existence. This universal energetic connection that we all share, explains how our intentions, healing thoughts, and prayers can connect us energetically to another person's mind and consciousness in order to send healing energy. The human body is made up of cells containing energy. These cells are made up of molecules, which are made up of atoms containing protons, neutrons and electrons. Atoms are made up of subatomic particles that are considered pure energy. Therefore, we are pure energy moving in waves with no boundaries, neither in space nor in time. This energy field is in everything that exists and has existed and is what connects us.

> For every action there is an equal and opposite reaction.
> ~ Newton's third law of motion

Energy allows us to accomplish what we need to. As we get older, energy becomes a valuable commodity as our cells can face an energy crisis. We have all experienced low energy and fatigue, wondering how we are going to accomplish what we need to do. This happens when there is a disruption of energy production in our mitochondria (the powerhouse of our cells), leading to reduced cellular energy and affecting the cell's ability to function properly, heal and regenerate.

I have combined Soul 7's Mindful Healing Technologies to help renew energy fields and rebalance any cellular dysfunction. This improves circulation that in turn brings more oxygen and nutrients to our cells. One of the technologies that we use is Pulsed Electromagnetic Field Therapy (PEMF). We use PEMF energy in alignment with the earth's geomagnetic and Schumann resonance to ignite our client's cellular energy. We have a mind-body-earth connection and our cells resonate to this healing frequency. "Using earth inspired PEMF therapy is like hooking up our hundred trillion cells to microscopic jumper cables, giving them a full charge. PEMF literally "jump-starts" the healing process in the body at the cellular level."[3]

Our thoughts and emotions have an electromagnetic frequency that affects every cell in our body. Be mindful of what you think because your cells are listening! Thoughts are waves of energy and the thoughts that occupy your mind is where your energy is flowing. The lower frequency waves, or thoughts, are based on fear and they create feelings of limitation, separation, and powerlessness. The higher frequency waves are based on love, acceptance, unity, faith, trust and feeling connected. Love transcends all other feelings and emotions. It is the energy that heals us. When we habitually experience repeated negative, low frequency thoughts and emotions, the energy tends to stagnate, congeal, and cause blockages, depleting us of energy. It is important to become aware of negative thought patterns and identify the source of what is causing the fear. Fear lets you know that you believe in a reality that is not aligned with your higher self. Over time, if not resolved, it leads to physical blockages causing disease.

Our PEMF technology can eliminate energy blockages caused by negative emotions while increasing awareness. By becoming aware of your thoughts, you can choose to change them. Decide what your new preferred reality is and adopt it by feeling it and breathing it in. You are now able to shift the fear into trust. A simple analogy to explain this is a radio, if you don't like the station you are listening to you can select a different channel. The other stations already exist, and at any time you have the option to choose another one. All possible versions of your reality exist simultaneously, all you have to do is select it and allow it in.

> Our level of consciousness is what creates our reality.
> Natural forces within us are the true healers of disease.
> ~ Hippocrates

Our bodies are electric and our cells need energy to function and nothing can happen without an electromagnetic exchange between cells. Our nervous system produces electrical energy and is sensitive to the other energies that come into its range. It responds to the electromagnetic fields produced by the hearts of the people around us. Our blood transports chemical energy and our mitochondria generate Adenosine Triphosphate (ATP), the energy necessary to sustain life. ATP transports chemical energy within our cells, regulating cell metabolism. It is interesting to note that our body creates almost twenty times more energy during exercise. PEMF therapy assists in the creation of ATP, and more energy means more vitality. Each heartbeat generates electromagnetic waves in all of our blood vessels, stimulating our tissues and communicating information to our brain and throughout our entire body. Our heart generates a powerful and extensive rhythmic electromagnetic field that permeates every cell in our body. Our hearts field is sixty times greater in amplitude, compared to the electromagnetic field produced by our brain and extends out in all directions in the space around us.[2] In fact, studies have shown that we have a detectable magnetic field that extends fifteen feet.[3] When we are close to someone, our energy fields interact and connect and we can even be influenced by their mood.

Our brain cells need a lot of energy to communicate with each other and with other parts of our body. Brain waves are generated by neurons, and communicate with each other through electrical charges. The electrical activity of our brain can be measured and seen by an EEG (electroencephalogram). There are four basic frequencies that our brain emits. Ranging from the most activity to the least activity are Beta, Alpha, Theta and Delta waves. These frequencies are the rate at which electrical charges move through the neurons. Delta waves are about 4 cycles per second and create deep relaxation and sleep, whereas, Beta brain waves are about 15 cycles per second and represent a heightened mental activity and an intense state of alertness. Beta waves are associated with lower frequency thoughts and emotions because we tend to be focused on the external. In Delta, the lower brain waves, we tend to be focused inwardly and are more centered and calm in our thoughts and emotions and in this state it is easier to change our perceptions. PEMF technology can help you access this frequency to help balance your mood, enhance clarity and give you a renewed sense of purpose and belonging.

Our muscle fibers need energy to help us move and maintain our posture. We derive metabolic energy from the food we eat, which is transferred to us through digestion. Food either gives us energy or depletes us of it depending on whether the food has been altered or processed. Our bodies are electric by nature and nothing can happen without the electromagnetic exchanges between our cells.

In order to become a generator of our own destiny, we need to keep our mind/body connection healthy. The earth creates magnetic fields that we resonate with and need in order to be healthy. As you can see, everything is energy and all energy is electromagnetic in nature. If we were to become isolated from these waves it would impair our mental capacity and lead to physical symptoms of disease. When we are deprived of sunlight we become chronically depressed. All of the cells in our body communicate via electromagnetic frequencies. Even viruses and bacteria resonate on a specific frequency.

In 1950, Dr. Royal Rife subjected bacteria and viruses to energetic wave frequencies that destroyed them. He documented destructive resonance frequencies for fifteen bacteria and viruses.[4] PEMF technology not only delivers the therapeutic effects of PEMF but can also read your electromagnetic signature and then prescribe healing PEMF wavelengths through pulsed biofeedback. It raises the electrical potential of our tissues that are in a weakened state, and restores them. It can also be used to destroy parasites and bacteria. PEMF technology can diagnose and send healing frequencies without side effects, while promoting a relaxed state. It has been approved by Health Canada. It is safe and noninvasive, improves circulation to help remove lymphatic congestion and aids in wound healing, bone re-growth, and pain relief. In combination with other Mindful Healing Technologies, PEMF therapy jump-starts the healing process allowing you to fulfill The Healing Option you deserve.

---

[1] PEMF, The 5th Element of Health, Bryant A. Meyers, © 2014, Bryant A. Meyers
[2] http://www.lumennatura.com/2012/03/29/hearts-consciousness-body-as-ultra-sensitive-antenna/
[3] PEMF, The 5th Element of Health, Bryant, A. Meyers, © 2014, Bryant A. Meyers
[4] http://rifevideos.com/dr_rife_and_cancer_a_realistic_view.html

Chapter 5

Technology:
The Catalyst to Self-Healing

> In every culture and in every medical tradition before ours, healing was accomplished by moving energy.
>
> ~ AlbertSzent-Gyorgyi
>
> Health is an energy dance, the more you have the better you feel.
>
> ~ Bryant A. Meyers

We are electro-magnetic Beings. Our bodies resonate with measurable energy. When properly flowing, our body is designed to heal itself. Our body's informational field has within it the blueprint for perfect health, we just need to get out of our own way and give the body what it needs. A wise man once said, "We are our own worst enemies." When we continuously think or accept negative thoughts and feelings about ourselves it causes a disruption in the flow of energy, which can affect the vitality and function of our cells and organs. The health of our body is dependent on the health of our cells communicating and functioning optimally, creating billions of reactions every second.

When we are feeling negative, hopeless, or in despair our body is vibrating at a lower frequency, making us more vulnerable to disease. According to Dr. Robert O. Becker, the health of our body can be determined by its frequency. Laughter and happiness raise our body's frequency, keeping us healthy and protecting us from disease. All of our organs resonate within a specific frequency range in order to be healthy. Colds, flues and diseases resonate on a lower frequency. Tropical fresh fruit has the highest electrical frequency because it is exposed to the most sunlight or life force energy, whereas processed foods don't even register a measurable frequency. Think about how you feel after you eat, do you feel energized or lethargic? We want to keep our bodies resonating on a higher energy frequency that is synchronized with the earth. Frequency is the key to our health and is the carrier of energy and information that our body needs in order to heal.

Have you ever noticed that you feel calmer and more at peace when you are in nature? That's because we have a mind-body-earth connection and we are dependent on the earth's frequencies. When you are in nature your body tunes into this frequency and you end up feeling relaxed and more at peace. In this state, our immune system is happy and healthy. All of the technologies at Soul 7, including the electro-magnetized water, are aligned to the earth's healing frequency known as the Schumann Resonance.

Every cell and organ in our body absorbs and emits sound and resonates with a particle frequency and color. Everything, including YOU, is in a constant state of vibration and the most elemental vibration is sound. We can use sound to heal our body.

Broadcasting the right frequency can help open your heart, prompt peace, and hasten healing. We all have felt the impact that music has on our brain and body. Our Neural Muscular Vibration technology uses the multi-frequency acoustic vibrations generated by specially composed music to facilitate healing at a neuro-muscular level. Every note and sound being generated has been deliberately composed to transmit healing muscular and mental commands through the sympathetic and parasympathetic nervous systems allowing for mental and physical balance.

> Sound is the carrier of consciousness taking you to places you have never been.
>
> ~ David Hulse

Since ancient times, sound has been used intuitively to enhance altered states of consciousness. Sound frequencies from singing bowls, bells, cymbals, drums, meditation gongs and chanting can correct disharmonies that cause imbalances in our body. Sound can realign our energy centers, often referred to as Chakras, to their correct resonant frequencies. Our first experience with sound is in our mother's womb. We are floating freely in the warm amniotic fluid, similar to a sensory deprivation chamber. Picking up sound and the electromagnetic healing vibrations of our mother's heart gives us what we need in order to develop and thrive.

Another technology that I have found to be extremely effective for healing is Brainwave Entrainment. Using isochronic tones and binaural beats, the technology induces states of consciousness designed to help relieve psychological stress and stabilize emotions to facilitate healing. This technology delivers rhythmic sensory stimulations such as pulses of sound or light to modulate our brainwave frequencies to induce a healing state of awareness. We combine this mind-activation technology with Soul 7's custom designed guided visualizations for maximum healing results.

You probably have never heard of anyone with heart cancer. The heart is warm due to its high blood circulation and oxygen levels. It also has the highest voltage or electrical energy of all the cells in our body. Cancer has been shown to have the lowest cellular energy and lives in a low oxygen environment. We now know that chronic illnesses have a diminished cellular voltage.[1] Dr. Katsunari Nishihara believes that a low core body temperature weakens our cells by damaging the mitochondria. Once the mitochondria—the powerhouse of the cell, is damaged, its cellular energy diminishes because it is not functioning optimally. Ninety percent of our energy is produced by the mitochondria via ATP (the energy currency of our cell). When your cells are producing energy you are healthy, if the cellular voltage drops you get sick. Chronic stress and suppressing emotions can also lower our body's core temperature affecting the mitochondria of our cells. Interestingly, when the body temperature decreases we are more prone to depression and other psychological abnormalities.[2] As the body's core temperature decreases all cellular energy also decreases. According to Dr. Nishihara, the optimal body temperature is 100 degrees F, as it helps in boosting immunity to fight infectious diseases. When our body temperature decreases our lymph stagnates and is not removing toxins efficiently.

In order to raise your core temperature Dr. Nishihara suggests eating hot foods, drinking only warm liquids, practicing deep breathing to reduce stress and exercising. Proper diet with an emphasis on chewing food and getting enough sun exposure and restful sleep are also important. There are herbal products available that can increase your core temperature. Getting a massage with therapeutic essential oils can improve the circulation in your body. Wearing amethyst on your body or lying on an amethyst infra-red heated mat will improve circulation and restore your core body temperature with the infrared rays and negatively charged ions emitting from the amethyst crystals. According to a study published in Science Daily, scientists from the National University of Singapore have found that it is possible for core body temperature to be controlled by the brain. They found that we are able to increase our core body temperature using certain meditation techniques along with guided mental imagery.[3]

Energy balancing therapy boosts the immune system by raising our body's frequency and core temperature. Pulsed Electro Magnetic Field Therapy (PEMF) uses pure copper current loops that are closely aligned to the earth's magnetic field. Our body resonates and recharges and is able to regenerate at this healing frequency, also known as the Schumann Resonance. It induces microcurrents in our cells and creates energy, healing our tissues and cells. Our brain waves regulate our nervous system and the earth's frequency is similar to the Alpha brainwave state that allows us to deeply relax. During this relaxation state we are able to let go of our habitual holding patterns of where we tend to carry the majority of our stress in our body. This allows our body's self-healing mechanisms to address the areas that are unbalanced.

Keeping the voltage of our cells charged within its healthy range keeps us healthy and vibrant. Our PEMF technology recharges our batteries, so to speak, by increasing the ATP production in the mitochondria of our cells. ATP is the energy currency in our cells because it is the energy that drives all of our biological processes including, immunity, respiration, circulation, and organ function to movement. PEMF therapy opens all the channels and pathways for all the essential elements needed to create energy in our mitochondria. PEMF helps with inflammation and edema (swelling) by restoring the sodium and potassium exchange within our cells. This leads to pain reduction and increased wound and bone healing. At my Soul 7 Wellness Centre, we use PEMF technology, combined with Biofeedback, to directly target the energy blockage causing the pain or dysfunction to help clients heal faster. By balancing the body's energy in a gentle way we can promote muscle relaxation and increased energy generation to promote accelerated healing.

Our Mindful Healing Technologies are combined to synergistically increase energy flow by promoting blood circulation and releasing energy blockage. The result is restored and regenerated energy. PEMF and the other therapies offered at Soul 7 not only recharge the body at the cellular level they also create a state of deep relaxation. Our PEMF therapy opens all the channels and pathways for essential elements needed to create the healing energy within ourselves.

According to Bryan A. Meyers in the book, *PEMF – The 5th Element of Health*, the top eight benefits of PEMF therapy are:

1. Stronger bones
2. Increased endorphins and pain relief
3. Better sleep by stimulating the production of melatonin
4. More energy ATP
5. Better oxygenation and circulation
6. Improved immunity and lymphatic circulation
7. Relaxation and stress reduction
8. Nerve and tissue regeneration

One of the other exciting benefits of our PEMF therapy is increased blood flow and nitric oxide production. This means better circulation and an enhanced sex life! The body knows how to heal itself, it just needs the essential building blocks including pure filtered water, organic fruits, sprouts and green leafy and colorful vegetables, sunlight, oxygen, and the earth's PEMFs. Our PEMF technology supplies the energy needed and opens the channels that transport all of these essential elements of life into your cells.

At the end of the day, I believe that every person has the ability to heal. In my healing travels since Jayne's passing, I have discovered technologies (which I call Mindful Healing Technologies) that can help the healer within each of us discover our personal Healing Option. That is my wish for you and my mission for Soul 7.

---

[1] PEMF, the 5th element
[2] http://davidjernigan.blogspot.ca/2012/11/cancer-and-low-body-temperature.html
[3] http://www.sciencedaily.com/releases/2013/04/130408084858.htm

Chapter 6
Renew and Rebalance

- Are you ready to experience pain free living?

Pain is a universal human experience. Whether it's emotional, mental or physical, pain is something that has touched all of our lives. Pain can come to us for various reasons and helps us expand and grow, by creating a desire for change. Why is it that we need to go through pain and suffering in order to make changes? Wouldn't it be easier to take a different route?

- Where is your pain?

Do you currently suffer from back pain, fibromyalgia, osteoarthritis, chronic pain, an acute sports injury or do you wake up in the morning feeling stiff? We have all had experiences with random or lingering aches and pains. It is inevitable that at some point in your life you will have a muscle strain injury from weight training, tennis, running, cycling, lifting a heavy object, stress, overstretching in yoga or even walking. Studies show that one out of five Canadians and three out of five older adults suffer from some form of chronic pain.[1]

Pain can also present itself as knots in your shoulders triggered by stress. Knots are the points within the muscle where the fibers are contracted and unable to release. Some knots can actively refer pain along your neural pathways, causing pain and contraction in another area. They affect our circulatory systems ability to bring much needed oxygenated blood and nutrients to our cells and to remove toxins from those areas. Over time, debris can accumulate and block our body's energy flow, preventing communication between our cells, resulting in physical illness.

Did you know that suppressed emotions could be expressed in your body as physical ailments, unexplained pain, numbness, inflexibility and even loss of movement? Disharmony appears in our mind before appearing in our body, presenting itself as a symptom. This is a sign that something is amiss, and needs our attention. Most of us cover up the symptoms or "messages" our body is trying to tell us, by taking some form of pain medication. We go about our daily lives until the medication wears off and the symptoms present themselves again, and then we repeat the cycle, never getting to the root cause.

- Why not address the source of your pain once and for all?

In my research to find Soul 7's healing technologies, I have looked for modalities that get at the root cause. I have found that with the right combination of therapies, recovery can be achieved without pills or surgery. For example, PEMF electromagnetic stimulation can help in the treatment of injuries as well as in speeding up regeneration of connective, nerve and wound tissue. There are also protocols for chronic pain, acute pain and inflammation. The technology uses biofeedback to locate the blockage in your body and then generates the appropriate wavelength to restore balance. This is done by sending out healing frequencies while stimulating acupuncture points along the meridians. The meridians are channels that conduct energy throughout the body like an intricate highway system, running through all of our major body systems. If a meridian's energy is obstructed or the energy is moving too fast or too slow, the system it is linked to is jeopardized and the affected organs will not function normally. This is how disease can occur.

Acupuncture points are tiny pools of energy that run along the meridians. Each point has a specific function, in relation to its specific organ system. There are approximately 2,000 different acupuncture points that lie along the body's meridians. The strongest points tend to be at the ends of the meridians, in the toes, ankles, knees, fingers, wrists and elbows. Very often a symptom showing up in one part of the body can be alleviated by stimulating an acupuncture point that is located in a completely different and opposite area of the body. This happens because the point that is being stimulated lies on a meridian that corresponds with an affected organ or tissue, and the energy of that specific acupuncture point can be transmitted along the meridian's path to the area in need of healing.

Mindful Healing Technologies open the meridians and transfers healing frequencies by stimulating acupuncture points. This releases any blockages and increases energy flow. It balances both the mind and body and helps you become more in tune with your inner guide. The healing benefits include stress reduction, relaxation, better sleep quality and increased immune function. Treatments can help bring about inner peace and harmony while balancing emotions. This mental balance also enhances learning, memory and mental clarity. On the physical level, Treatments help to relieve pain and speed up the recovery process. The Mindful Healing Technologies that I have discovered and combined can reverse the degenerative effects of disease and reduce pain and inflammation. Getting at the root cause can translate into lasting results.

We are living in a time where many of us expect to have health issues when we reach a certain age, and shrug off aches and pains as age related. It's as though we have a pebble in our shoe and instead of trying to remove it, we find ways to walk around with it. Many people expect that they will inevitably be on some form of medication, and unfortunately our medical model is focused on illness rather than wellness. The pharmaceutical industry sells us billions of pain relief pills in all different shapes and sizes. The drug companies compete for control of this multibillion-dollar pain drug market with continuous advertising, and as a result, we all have some form of pain relief medication in our medicine cabinets.

We are the sum total of our life experiences. Aging is not something that happens on our sixty-fifth birthday. Aging well is dependent on how your body heals itself throughout your lifetime. Aging may be inevitable but the rate of aging is not. The choices you make and the thoughts you think have an impact on the health of your body, and daily stresses have a direct impact on your health.

> People don't grow old. When they stop growing, they become old.
>
> ~ Author Unknown

As our bodies age it is harder for our cells to adapt to stress. We have been exposed to a lifetime of damaging agents creating free radical damage adversely affecting our cellular functions. We eat a higher sodium meal and end up with bags under our eyes and swollen hands or feet as a result. This cellular edema (swelling) is caused by an impaired ion exchange within our cells. We may have even noticed declining energy levels. The Mindful Healing Technologies I have found increase the body's supply of circulating electrons, which are potent antioxidants. It improves circulation and opens channels in our cell membranes allowing more nutrients and oxygen in and toxins and waste out, improving our overall energy and the look and feel of our skin. By correcting nutrient deficiencies, improving insomnia and treating the damaging effects of chronic stress our technologies produce lasting anti-aging benefits.

Combined with neural muscular vibration therapy, the Mindful Healing Technologies I have assembled can help you access a calm, meditative brain wave frequency of wellbeing and tranquility. At this frequency we have a heightened awareness and receptivity to create lasting changes in our body. Neural muscular vibration therapy increases serotonin and endorphins, improving our overall mood, making us feel happier and calm. As well, research is showing that guided visualization can cause immediate, measurable physiological changes in our body to help reduce and eliminate chronic pain and manage and reduce stress. Soul 7's technologies combine to unblock and balance the energy flow that helps the body's immune system achieve optimal health.

- So, what are energy blockages?

> When energy flows freely along the meridians, we are free from illness; if the energy is blocked, the pain follows.
>
> ~ Chinese Medicine

An energy blockage is caused by an accumulation of stagnant energy, stemming from unresolved conscious or unconscious life experiences that get stored in our tissues and create energy blockages, which lead to pain. The most common emotions we tend to hang on to are the negative ones such as fear, regret, anger or sadness. Even positive emotions like happiness can be a nostalgic memory linked to our past, which can keep us living in the past, while not being present in our lives. Despite these blockages, our body retains the memory of healthy energy flow. Once these blockages are stimulated by Soul 7's energy balancing technology, your body will be able to restore the energy flow back to its original pattern. Opening an energy blockage allows chemical waste to be removed and brings oxygenated blood flow and nutrients to our cells.

Your body has an innate healing wisdom and by releasing energy blockages it can create harmony and energy flow, leading to pain relief and greater balance within your body. Soul 7's Mindful Healing Technologies syner-gistically combine to communicate with your central nervous system, helping to release tension and accumulated stress, clearing the way for your body's own healing wisdom to take effect.

The technology activates what is already known within the body and helps us access it. One of the problems with western medicine and some alternative medicine is that they tend to add energy into sustaining the unwanted health condition. By devoting more attention to its existence and making our 'health conditions' more self-aware, it reinforces their strength. My goal at Soul 7 is to get to the source of any disharmony, pain or disease occurring within the body, by improving the overall health of the cells and by rebalancing and repairing any cellular dysfunction that may be occurring. Mindful Healing Technologies help us become more self-aware by reminding us that our body has an innate healing potential and all we have to do is give our body what it needs in order for it to find The Healing Option right for you.

---

[1] Mailis-Gagnon, A. (2010). The hurting numbers. Action Ontario Pain Advocacy Newsletter, 2(1), 5.

Chapter 7

Healthy Practices

We all have responsibilities and commitments, but we can choose to approach them in a more positive light. As you embark on your personal healing journey, here are some healthy practices that I have found helpful on my own journey.

Begin by finding joy in your everyday existence and making peace with what is. Spend some time alone; meditate, write, sketch, do some yoga or simply sit quietly for a few minutes each day and do absolutely nothing. There is an Italian phrase "Dolce Far Niente" which means the sweetness of doing nothing. Learn to embrace your down time!

When our internal environment is healthy, it naturally provides neurotransmitters and hormones to help us "feel good" and to overcome stressful situations. When those resources are not accessible and we don't have the nutritional resources to draw from, our natural instinct is to find them externally in order to seek relief from pain. Unfortunately, unhealthy junk food full of fat and chemical additives, too much sugar, salt, caffeine and alcohol are easier and more accessible. This just sets you up for addictions, creating a vicious cycle. The key to keeping yourself healthy and balanced is to give your body what it needs to thrive. Our body needs organic fruits and vegetables in abundance, filtered water, sunlight, fresh air, plenty of sleep, exercise and the earth's PEMFs.

Reconnecting to the earth by walking barefoot has many powerful effects on your wellbeing and can help you on your healing journey. We resonate with the earth's frequency, helping us feel calm and more at peace and at the same time energizing our body. Grounding yourself by touching the earth's surface directly allows the energy to be transferred into your skin, creating a barrier against free radical damage. We are bombarded with electrosmog from computers, cell phones, cell towers and from the decline in the earth's magnetic field. The Earth's energy helps with stress reduction and the promotion of sleep, helping to speed up the healing process. Take time each day to be in nature. In the summer, take your shoes off and walk barefoot through the grass. Do Tai Chi in the park, take up gardening, camping and hiking or go for a walk, anything that brings you back to nature. Get at least half an hour of natural sunlight everyday by being outdoors.

> We are a part of nature, not apart from nature.
>
> ~ Author Unknown

The importance of good digestion can oftentimes be overlooked. The majority of our immune function resides in our gut, so it is crucial that we keep our entire gastrointestinal tract clean and regular. This can be done by eating a wholesome, fiber-rich diet of high vibrational living foods like fruits, sprouts and vegetables, and by drinking enough filtered water. Regular and healthy elimination is essential because we need a way of removing toxins from our bodies.

Our lymphatic system is our drainage system and works together with the immune system to destroy pathogens and to filter waste. When the lymph system becomes overburdened with toxins, parasites, mucous and metabolic wastes your lymph nodes will become enlarged and swollen. By keeping the energy flowing and the blood circulating, we are speeding up the healing process and increasing our immune function. Dry skin brushing, rebounding, infrared sauna and daily exercises such as Tai Chi are ways we can keep our lymphatic system healthy.

Dry skin brushing is a fantastic way to increase the circulation and lymphatic drainage of the skin. This practice helps shed dead skin cells and encourages cell renewal, which results in smoother and younger looking skin. It helps with muscle tone and gives you a more even distribution of fat deposits, thus reducing the appearance of cellulite. Dry skin brushing is best done before bathing. Always begin at the ankles and brush in gentle, upward, circular movements towards the heart. This is the direction that the lymphatic fluid flows. Alternating the temperature of the shower from hot to cold will further refresh the skin and stimulate blood circulation.

Infrared saunas and mats (we use them at Soul 7) help your body release toxins, including heavy metals and environmental chemicals. With infrared heat technology, you can lose weight, relax, relieve unwanted pain from inflammation, increase your circulation, and purify your skin. This is a great complementary tool to add to our Soul 7 programs as it can increase healing time and reduce overall stress levels.

Rebounding, also known as trampoline jumping, is a fun way to get healthy. Rebounding increases lymphatic drainage and immune function, improves digestion and increases circulation throughout the body. It will get your heart rate up and increase your endurance on a cellular level by increasing oxygenated blood flow, while improving both strength and balance.

Proper breathing is important in order to keep your mind and body healthy. Deep breathing techniques can help decrease stress levels by releasing any built up tension in the body, while having a calming effect on the mind. Deep breathing relieves anxiety by increasing endorphin production, thus relieving pain. Proper breathing techniques are important for good digestion and assimilation and a healthy immune system. Controlled breathing also strengthens and tones your abdominal muscles and improves your posture. I believe that proper breathing is so important to the healing process that I have instituted a Resonance Frequency Breathing (RFB) Program that uses biofeedback technology invented by one of the world's leading sport psychologists to measure each client's optimal breathing rate. Once you choose The Healing Option, you deserve to be treated like a world-class athlete. Not because you are one. Not because you will become one. But, because that's what it takes to achieve your optimal health.

Conclusion

Despite the loss of my wife and my own health challenges, my personal healing journey has led me to conclude that our body's natural inclination and wisdom is to always strive for health and balance. Our body has an innate wisdom and knows exactly what it needs in order to heal itself. The healer is within each of us. All we have to do is choose The Healing Option. Once we make that choice, we access a deep intuitive healing connection that will lead to our personal optimal health … which is what I wish for you.

InPeace,,

Bob Berman, Soul 7 Founder

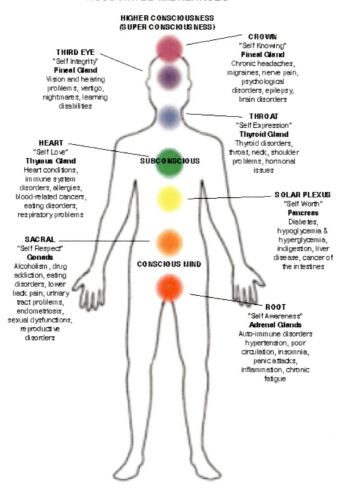

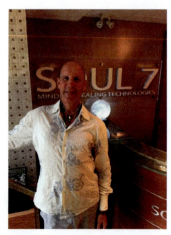

Bob Berman, Founder, Soul 7

Bob is the father of three amazing human beings and GrandBob to another. He loves humanity and cherishes Mother Earth. As Soul 7's Founder, Bob is grateful for the opportunity to further Soul 7's Mission by introducing people to and helping to optimize their innate ability to Self Heal, Mind, Body and Soul. He loves Physics and Metaphysics. For Bob's take on the *Quantum Mechanics of the Healing Process*, check out his very short essay by the same name.

If nothing else, he wants you to know that...

Love is the ultimate Healer...beginning with YOU.

Soul 7 Inc.

17 Yorkville Avenue

Toronto, Ontario M4W 1L1

416.847.6999 • 1.855.387.6857

E-mail: info@soul7.ca

Website: www.soul7.ca

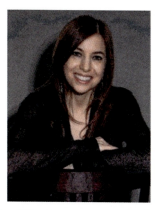

Ara Wiseman, RHN, RNCP, Author

Ara Wiseman is a leading nutritional expert, author, teacher and lecturer. Her thriving private practice is primarily focused on nutrition counseling for addictions, weight loss and gain, hormonal imbalances, cancer and heart disease. Ara teaches nutrition at the Transformational Arts College in Toronto, and has written and published the following books: *Feed Your Body, Feed Your Soul* (2010, Maiden Tree Media), *Skin Deep, How to Diminish Cellulite* (2012), *A Smoother You* (2014, Maiden Tree Media) and *The Secrets to Anti-Aging* to be released February 2015.

Ara lives in Toronto and can be reached at:
Tel: 416.876.8155
E-mail: info@arawiseman.com
Website: www.arawiseman.com

Resources/Scientific Journals

1. "Beneficial effects of electromagnetic fields", Bassett C. (Bioelectric Research Center, Columbia University, NY, 1993).
   A wide variety of musculoskeletal disorders have been treated successfully through PEMF therapy including nerve regeneration, wound healing, skin graft healing, diabetes, heart attack and stroke, among other conditions. There have also been possible benefits in controlling malignancy of cancer cells.
   http://onlinelibrary.wiley.com/doi/10.1002/jcb.2400510402/abstract

2. "Treating cancer with amplitude-modulated electromagnetic fields: a potential paradigm shift, again?", Blackman (British Journal of Cancer, 2012).
   Research shows that PEMF can be selective in treating cancer cells. Reduced growth rate was observed for tumor cells exposed to tissue-specific AM-EMF, but there was no change in the growth rate of normal cells derived from the same tissue type.
   http://www.nature.com/bjc/journal/v106/n2/full/bjc2011576a.html

3. "Cancer cell proliferation is inhibited by specific modulation frequencies", Zimmerman et al. (British Journal of Cancer, 2012).
   Researchers have demonstrated that small doses of electromagnetism can shrink liver and breast cancer cells without harming surrounding tissues.
   http://www.nature.com/bjc/journal/v106/n2/pdf/bjc2011523a.pdf

4. "Treatment of advanced hepatocellular carcinoma with very low levels of amplitude-modulated electromagnetic fields" Zimmerman et al. (British Journal of Cancer, 2011
   Researchers were able to slow tumor growth in some HCC patients by treating them with low-level electromagnetic fields on a regular basis. After 6 months of treatment, tumor growth in several patients had stabilized with no negative side effects.
   http://www.nature.com/bjc/journal/v105/n5/abs/bjc2011292a.html

5. "Differential sensitivities of malignant and normal skin cells to nanosecond pulsed electric fields," Yang W et al. (University of Southern California, Los Angeles, CA, 2011).
   Research concluded that in paired tumor and normal skin cell lines, the response of the tumor cells to nanoelectropulse exposure is stronger than the response of normal cells, indicating the potential for selectivity in therapeutic applications.
   http://www.ncbi.nlm.nih.gov/pubmed/21517135

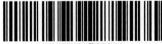

Made in the USA
Columbia, SC
14 September 2018